ARTHRITIS FRIENDLY WORKOUTS

Fitness Routines That Cater to Individuals with Arthritis, Focusing on Joint-Friendly Exercises.

Basil U.

COPYRIGHT

TABLE OF CONTENTS

ABOUT THE BOOK

Arthritis affects millions of individuals worldwide, and its impact can be profound—limiting mobility, reducing quality of life, and instilling fear of physical activity. Yet, this book aims to challenge the misconceptions surrounding exercise for those living with arthritis. "Arthritis-Friendly Workouts" is designed to be a comprehensive guide for anyone seeking to maintain an active lifestyle while managing the challenges of this condition. With a focus on joint-friendly exercises, this book provides practical advice, real-life stories, and adaptable workout routines tailored to the unique needs of individuals with arthritis.

Understanding Arthritis

Arthritis is not a single disease but a term encompassing over 100 different conditions that affect the joints, with osteoarthritis and rheumatoid arthritis being the most common types. These conditions can lead to inflammation, pain, and stiffness, which can make physical activity seem daunting or even impossible. However, staying active is crucial for maintaining joint function and overall health. This book delves into the science of arthritis, explaining how it affects the body and why exercise should be an integral part of arthritis management.

The Importance of Exercise

Despite the common belief that exercise may exacerbate joint pain, research shows that regular physical activity can significantly reduce pain and improve function for individuals with arthritis. This book emphasizes the benefits of exercise, highlighting how it can help manage weight, improve mood, boost cardiovascular health, and enhance flexibility. Each chapter is infused with motivational insights and success stories from individuals who have successfully integrated exercise into their lives, proving that a fulfilling and active lifestyle is within reach.

Comprehensive, Adaptable Workouts

"Arthritis-Friendly Workouts" offers a diverse range of low-impact exercises specifically designed to cater to the needs of those with joint issues. From warm-up routines and stretching techniques to aerobic workouts, strength training, and flexibility exercises, each section provides clear instructions and modifications to ensure safety and effectiveness. The book recognizes that no two journeys are the same, which is why it encourages readers to personalize their fitness plans based on their specific type of arthritis and individual capabilities.

 Practical Guidance and Support

Throughout the book, readers will find essential tips for preparing for workouts, selecting appropriate equipment, and establishing a consistent exercise routine. Special attention is given to listening to one's body and understanding the difference between discomfort and pain, which is critical for preventing injury. The author shares strategies for modifying exercises based on the type of arthritis, allowing individuals to adapt their workouts as needed.

Building a Supportive Community

Living with arthritis can often feel isolating, but this book underscores the importance of community and connection. By joining arthritis-friendly fitness classes and support groups, individuals can share their experiences, challenges, and triumphs, fostering motivation and accountability. The book encourages readers to seek out resources and communities that align with their fitness goals, ensuring they never feel alone on their journey.

Nutrition and Lifestyle Tips

In addition to exercise, the book addresses the role of nutrition and lifestyle in managing arthritis. Readers will discover how certain foods can promote joint health, reduce inflammation, and help manage weight—an essential factor for reducing stress on the joints. The book also provides practical tips for creating a daily routine that incorporates movement, ensuring that physical activity becomes a seamless part of life rather than a chore.

A Path Toward Empowerment

Ultimately, "Arthritis-Friendly Workouts" is about empowerment. It invites readers to embrace a positive mindset and redefine their understanding of fitness. Each chapter is written in modern, accessible language, offering practical advice intertwined with personal anecdotes that resonate with the reader's journey. The goal is to inspire individuals to see exercise not as a punishment or a source of pain but as a powerful tool for reclaiming their lives and achieving their fitness aspirations.

This book is more than just a fitness manual; it is a guide to living a vibrant, active life despite arthritis. With compassion, expertise, and a deep understanding of the unique challenges faced by individuals with this condition, "Arthritis-Friendly Workouts" stands as a beacon of hope and encouragement. Whether you are newly diagnosed or have been managing arthritis for years, this book is your companion on the journey to finding joy in movement and cultivating a lifestyle that prioritizes health, wellness, and resilience.

INTRODUCTION

Arthritis is more than just a single condition; it's an umbrella term that encompasses over a hundred different diseases, the most common being osteoarthritis and rheumatoid arthritis. Each type presents its unique challenges, primarily affecting the joints, leading to pain, stiffness, and reduced mobility. For millions, these symptoms can feel like an insurmountable barrier to living an active and fulfilling life. However, understanding arthritis is the first step toward reclaiming that life. By recognizing how this condition impact's joint function and overall movement, individuals can begin to navigate their exercise journey more effectively.

Despite the discomfort that arthritis can bring, remaining physically active is crucial. Movement may seem counterintuitive when faced with joint pain, yet studies show that engaging in regular exercise can significantly improve joint function and alleviate stiffness. The key lies in choosing the right kinds of exercises—those that are gentle and joint-friendly. By doing so, individuals not only combat pain but also enhance their overall well-being, bolstering their mood and quality of life.

Unfortunately, many myths surrounding exercise and arthritis persist. Some believe that physical activity will worsen their condition, while others think they should avoid movement altogether. These misconceptions can lead to a sedentary lifestyle, which is often more detrimental than the condition itself. Inactivity can exacerbate pain, reduce flexibility, and lead to further complications, such as weight gain and decreased cardiovascular health. By shedding light on these misconceptions, we aim to empower readers to embrace a more active lifestyle, despite their arthritis.

In this book, we will explore the myriad benefits of exercise for those living with arthritis. From reducing pain and stiffness to improving mental health, the advantages of regular physical activity are profound. We'll also discuss what happens when movement is neglected, emphasizing the importance of incorporating exercise into daily routines.

Written in a modern, accessible style, this book combines practical advice with relatable anecdotes and success stories, creating a narrative that engages and inspires. Our goal is to equip readers with the knowledge and tools necessary to develop arthritis-friendly workout routines, ensuring they can enjoy an active, healthy life, regardless of their condition. Together, let's embark on a journey toward better joint health and enhanced well-being through movement.

CHAPTER 1

PREPARING FOR AN ARTHRITIS-FRIENDLY WORKOUT

Embarking on a fitness journey when you have arthritis requires careful preparation and thoughtful consideration. The right foundation can make all the difference in ensuring your exercise experience is safe, enjoyable, and effective. In this chapter, we'll explore the essential steps to prepare for an arthritis-friendly workout, emphasizing the importance of professional guidance and the appropriate gear.

Consulting Your Doctor or Physiotherapist

Before diving into any fitness program, the first and most critical step is to consult your healthcare provider. Each person's experience with arthritis is unique, influenced by the type of arthritis, its severity, and individual health circumstances. A doctor or physiotherapist can provide valuable insights tailored to your specific condition, helping you identify which exercises are safe and beneficial.

For instance, when Mary, a 62-year-old woman with osteoarthritis in her knees, approached her doctor about exercise, she was initially apprehensive. Her doctor evaluated her condition and, recognizing her desire to stay active, recommended a mix of low-impact aerobics and strength training that would help support her joints without causing further strain. This personalized guidance not only gave Mary the confidence to start exercising but also helped her avoid movements that could exacerbate her condition.

Creating a personalized workout plan is essential. This plan should consider your current fitness level, joint health, and any other underlying health issues. A physiotherapist can help you develop a program that gradually increases in intensity, ensuring you build strength and flexibility without overdoing it. This tailored approach will allow you to stay engaged and motivated, making your fitness journey more sustainable and enjoyable.

Selecting the Right Equipment and Gear

Once you've consulted with your healthcare provider and established a workout plan, the next step is to invest in the right equipment and gear. Proper footwear plays a pivotal role in protecting your joints and enhancing your exercise experience. Look for shoes that offer good arch support, cushioning, and stability. Avoid flat-soled shoes or those that lack adequate support, as they can increase the risk of injury and joint strain.

Consider how footwear impacted James, a retired firefighter who had struggled with rheumatoid arthritis for years. After switching to shoes designed specifically for those with arthritis, he noticed a significant difference in his comfort level during workouts. With improved support, he could engage in walking and light jogging without the sharp pains he previously experienced.

In addition to shoes, incorporating exercise props can greatly benefit your workout routine. Resistance bands and light weights are excellent options for building strength without putting excessive pressure on your joints. These tools are versatile and can be adjusted based on your fitness level, allowing for gradual progress. For example, Lisa, a

55-year-old living with arthritis, began using resistance bands during her strength training sessions. Initially, she used a light resistance band, which helped her strengthen her muscles without feeling overwhelmed. Over time, she gradually increased the resistance, leading to improved strength and stability in her joints.

Furthermore, clothing choices matter when it comes to comfort and mobility. Opt for breathable, stretchy fabrics that allow for freedom of movement. Avoid clothing that is too tight or restrictive, as it can hinder your range of motion. Mary discovered the joy of wearing moisture-wicking fabrics during her workouts, which helped her stay comfortable and focused on her exercises instead of feeling weighed down by her clothing.

If you participate in classes or workouts, consider layering your clothing. This way, you can easily adjust to changes in body temperature as you warm up and cool down. And don't forget about accessories like knee or wrist supports if you find they provide extra stability during workouts.

Getting Started: The First Steps

With professional guidance and the right gear in place, you're ready to embark on your fitness journey. Start with short sessions that emphasize warm-ups, gentle movements, and stretches. Listen to your body and monitor how it responds to each exercise. It's natural to feel some discomfort, but you should never feel sharp pain. Use your initial sessions to learn what works best for you and gradually build confidence.

As you become more comfortable, consider incorporating a mix of aerobic exercises, strength training, and flexibility work into your routine. For instance, you might start with a 10-minute walk, followed by some bodyweight exercises, and conclude with gentle stretching. Document your progress and adjust your plan as necessary, seeking feedback from your healthcare provider along the way.

Throughout this process, remember that patience is key. Progress may be slow at times, but every step you take is a step toward improved joint health and a more active lifestyle. Embrace the journey, celebrate small victories, and don't hesitate to lean on support systems, whether they be friends, family, or community groups.

Preparing for an arthritis-friendly workout is about more than just physical readiness; it involves a thoughtful approach to your health, gear, and overall mindset. By consulting healthcare professionals, selecting appropriate equipment, and embracing gradual progress, you'll set yourself up for success. Each workout will not only contribute to your physical health but also to your emotional well-being, empowering you to lead a more active, fulfilling life despite arthritis.

As you move forward, let this chapter serve as a foundation for your fitness journey—one that is informed, supported, and tailored to your unique needs. With the right preparation, you are not just managing your arthritis; you are taking an active role in your health and well-being.

CHAPTER 2

WARM-UP AND STRETCHING FOR JOINT HEALTH

As you embark on your fitness journey, the importance of warming up and stretching cannot be overstated. These practices are vital in preparing your body for exercise, particularly when you're living with arthritis. A proper warm-up routine can help lubricate your joints, reduce stiffness, and enhance your overall performance, while stretching improves flexibility and can alleviate pain. In this chapter, we'll explore effective warm-up techniques and safe stretching methods designed specifically for those with arthritis.

The Importance of Warming Up Before Exercise

Warming up is like prepping your car before a long drive; it's essential for a smooth journey. When you engage in warm-up exercises, your body gradually increases blood flow to the muscles and joints. This process raises the temperature of your muscles, making them more pliable and less prone to injury. For people with arthritis, this is particularly crucial. Warming up helps to lubricate the joints, easing stiffness and preparing them for movement.

Consider the experience of Tom, a 59-year-old who has battled osteoarthritis for several years. Initially, Tom would jump straight into his workouts, thinking he could save time. However, he soon found that without a warm-up, his joints felt stiff and painful, limiting his ability to complete his routines. After incorporating a warm-up into his regimen, Tom noticed a remarkable difference. He felt lighter, more agile, and his pain levels significantly decreased during his workouts.

So, what should a warm-up routine look like? A great starting point is gentle walking. This simple activity can be done indoors or outdoors and allows your heart rate to gradually increase. Aim for about 5 to 10 minutes of brisk walking, paying attention to your breath and movements. If you prefer, you can also use a stationary bike or elliptical machine for a low-impact option.

In addition to walking, consider including range-of-motion exercises in your warm-up. These movements help increase flexibility and prepare your joints for the work ahead. Here are a few recommendations:

1. **Arm Circles**: Stand or sit comfortably, extend your arms to the side, and make small circles. Gradually increase the size of the circles, then reverse the direction.

2. **Ankle Rolls**: While seated or standing, lift one foot off the ground and rotate your ankle in a circular motion. Repeat with the other ankle.

3. **Hip Swings**: Stand with your hands on your hips and gently swing one leg forward and backward, keeping your movements controlled. Switch legs after 10 swings.

These warm-up exercises can be tailored to your fitness level and can be performed at your own pace. The key is to listen to your body and focus on movements that feel comfortable.

Stretching for Flexibility and Reduced Pain

Once you've completed your warm-up, it's time to incorporate stretching into your routine. Stretching is crucial for maintaining flexibility, which can be compromised in individuals with arthritis. Regular stretching can reduce pain and enhance your range of motion, making daily activities easier and more enjoyable.

When it comes to stretching, safety should be your top priority. Always perform stretches slowly and gently, avoiding any movements that cause sharp pain. It's essential to focus on the major joints—knees, hips, hands, and shoulders—since these areas are often most affected by arthritis.

Let's delve into some safe stretching techniques:

1. Knee Stretch: While sitting on a chair, extend one leg straight in front of you, keeping your heel on the ground. Gently lean forward until you feel a stretch in your hamstrings. Hold for 15-30 seconds, then switch legs.

2. Hip Flexor Stretch: Stand with your feet shoulder-width apart. Take a step back with one leg, keeping the front knee bent and the back leg straight. You should feel a stretch in the front of your hip. Hold for 15-30 seconds, then switch sides.

3. Wrist and Finger Stretch: Extend one arm in front of you, palm facing up. With the other hand, gently pull back on the fingers, feeling the stretch in your wrist and forearm. Hold for 15-30 seconds and switch sides.

4. Shoulder Stretch: Bring one arm across your body at chest height and use the opposite hand to gently pull the arm closer to your chest. Hold for 15-30 seconds, then switch arms.

When considering stretching techniques, it's essential to distinguish between dynamic and static stretching. Dynamic stretching involves moving parts of your body through a full range of motion in a controlled manner. This type of stretching can be beneficial during warm-ups as it prepares your muscles for action.

On the other hand, static stretching, which involves holding a stretch for a prolonged period, is typically more beneficial during cooldowns or following your workout. This is especially relevant for arthritis sufferers, as static stretches can help alleviate tension and improve flexibility.

For instance, after completing her workout, Lisa incorporates static stretches focusing on her shoulders and hips. By holding each stretch for about 30 seconds, she finds that her muscles relax and her joint stiffness decreases, making her feel more comfortable throughout the day.

Warming up and stretching are integral components of an arthritis-friendly workout routine. By preparing your body for exercise, you can reduce the risk of injury, enhance your performance, and ultimately improve your overall quality of life. Incorporating gentle warm-up activities and safe stretching techniques tailored to your needs will ensure that you can move more freely and with less discomfort.

As you progress in your fitness journey, remember to listen to your body and adjust your routines accordingly. Each person's experience with arthritis is unique, so find what works best for you. By dedicating time to warm up and stretch, you're not just preparing your body for exercise; you're investing in your long-term health and well-being. Embrace these practices as part of your daily routine, and watch as they transform your relationship with movement, helping you lead a more active and fulfilling life.

CHAPTER 3

LOW-IMPACT AEROBIC EXERCISES

Aerobic exercise plays a crucial role in managing arthritis, offering a pathway to improved health and enhanced quality of life. For individuals living with this condition, finding suitable workouts that promote cardiovascular health without putting excessive strain on the joints is essential. In this chapter, we'll explore the benefits of low-impact aerobic exercises and highlight some of the most joint-friendly workouts available.

The Role of Aerobic Exercise in Managing Arthritis

Aerobic exercise is fundamental for those living with arthritis for several reasons. One of the primary benefits is its role in weight management. Excess weight can place additional pressure on already-stressed joints, particularly the knees and hips. By incorporating regular aerobic activity into your routine, you can help manage your weight, reducing strain on these critical areas and alleviating pain.

For example, Sarah, a 65-year-old grandmother with osteoarthritis, found that she was carrying more weight than she felt comfortable with. After starting a walking program, she not only shed some pounds but also noticed a significant reduction in her knee pain. Her experience illustrates how even small changes in weight can lead to meaningful improvements in joint comfort and mobility.

Aerobic exercise also boosts cardiovascular health, promoting overall well-being. Increased heart rate and improved circulation contribute to better oxygen delivery throughout the body, which is crucial for maintaining healthy tissues and joints. Moreover, regular aerobic activity can enhance mood and reduce anxiety, which are often exacerbated by chronic pain conditions. This connection between physical activity and mental health is essential for anyone dealing with arthritis, as it fosters a more positive outlook and encourages continued engagement in fitness.

Joint-Friendly Aerobic Workouts

Now that we've established the importance of aerobic exercise, let's explore specific low-impact workouts that can benefit individuals with arthritis.

Walking: The Simplest, Most Effective Workout for Arthritis

Walking is perhaps the most accessible and effective form of aerobic exercise for those with arthritis. It requires no special equipment and can be done almost anywhere. This simple activity not only helps manage weight but also improves cardiovascular health and enhances flexibility.

For those who may find walking outdoors challenging, consider walking indoors or utilizing a treadmill. You can start with short distances and gradually increase your time and pace as your body adapts. Jane, a 58-year-old who has struggled with rheumatoid arthritis, discovered that walking in her local mall allowed her to avoid harsh weather while enjoying the supportive environment. With the combination of gentle movement and social interaction, Jane felt encouraged to continue her fitness journey.

Swimming and Water Aerobics: The Benefits of Water for Joint Relief

Water-based exercises are another excellent option for arthritis sufferers. Swimming and water aerobics allow you to engage in cardiovascular activity with minimal impact on your joints. The buoyancy of water supports your body weight, reducing strain on your joints while providing resistance to enhance muscle strength.

Take the story of Michael, a 72-year-old retiree who found solace in his local swimming pool. Initially intimidated by the idea of swimming, he quickly learned that the water provided an environment where he could move freely without fear of injury. His water aerobics class became a highlight of his week, not only for the physical benefits but also for the social connection it fostered with fellow participants.

Cycling: How It Promotes Movement Without Straining the Knees

Cycling is another fantastic low-impact aerobics option, whether on a stationary bike or outdoors. It promotes movement and helps strengthen the leg muscles without putting excessive stress on the knees. This form of exercise is particularly appealing for those who enjoy the feeling of speed and movement.

For instance, Carla, a 60-year-old woman diagnosed with osteoarthritis, found that cycling allowed her to stay active without the jarring impact of walking or jogging. She started with short sessions on a stationary bike at home and gradually built her endurance, eventually joining a local cycling group. Not only did this new hobby boost her fitness level, but it also expanded her social circle, enhancing her quality of life.

Chair-Based Aerobics for Those with Limited Mobility

For individuals with limited mobility or those who find traditional aerobic exercises too challenging, chair-based aerobics can be a perfect solution. These workouts are designed to be performed while seated, providing a safe and effective way to engage in cardiovascular activity.

Chair-based aerobics can incorporate a variety of movements, such as seated marching, arm raises, and gentle twisting. Not only do these exercises promote cardiovascular health, but they also help improve flexibility and strength. For example, Tom, a 70-year-old man with severe arthritis in his hips, initially felt discouraged by his limitations. However, he discovered chair aerobics classes at his local community center. Through these classes, he learned that he could still engage in meaningful movement and connect with others, empowering him to take charge of his health.

Low-impact aerobic exercises are essential for managing arthritis effectively. By incorporating activities such as walking, swimming, cycling, and chair-based aerobics into your routine, you can promote weight management, enhance cardiovascular health, and improve your overall well-being.

As you explore these options, remember to listen to your body and adjust your activities to suit your individual needs. The journey to better health may come with its challenges, but with dedication and the right approach, you can find joy and fulfillment in movement. Whether you're taking your first steps or diving into water aerobics, know that every effort counts and contributes to a healthier, more active life. Embrace these low-impact workouts, and let them empower you on your journey to better joint health and overall wellness.

CHAPTER 4

STRENGTH TRAINING FOR ARTHRITIS

When it comes to managing arthritis, strength training may not be the first exercise that comes to mind. Yet, it plays an essential role in enhancing joint support and improving overall functionality. In this chapter, we'll discuss why strength training is crucial for individuals with arthritis, explore effective exercises targeting key joint areas, and outline best practices for safe training.

Why Strength Training is Essential for Joint Support

Strength training is vital for those living with arthritis, primarily because it builds muscle around the joints. Strong muscles act as stabilizers, helping to protect weakened joints from injury and reducing the strain placed upon them during daily activities. For instance, when the muscles around your knees are well-developed, they can absorb impact and minimize stress on the joint itself, leading to less pain and discomfort.

Consider the experience of Emma, a 64-year-old who has dealt with osteoarthritis in her knees for several years. Initially, she was hesitant to try strength training, fearing it might exacerbate her pain. However, after consulting with her physiotherapist, she learned that building muscle strength could actually relieve some of the pressure on her knees. Emma began a gradual strength training program, focusing on exercises that targeted her leg muscles, and soon noticed a remarkable improvement in her stability and overall comfort.

In addition to providing joint support, strength training is also crucial for preventing bone loss, which is particularly important as we age. Osteoporosis can be a concern for many individuals, especially those with arthritis. By engaging in strength exercises, you can promote bone density and help protect against fractures. Moreover, improved balance is another benefit of strength training, reducing the risk of falls—a significant concern for individuals with joint issues.

Strengthening Exercises for Key Joint Areas

Now that we understand the importance of strength training, let's explore specific exercises that can benefit individuals with arthritis. These exercises can be performed using body weight, light weights, or resistance bands, depending on your comfort level and physical abilities.

Bodyweight Exercises

1. Squats: Squats can help strengthen the muscles around your knees and hips. Start by standing with your feet shoulder-width apart. Lower your body as if you were going to sit back in a chair, keeping your weight in your heels and your back straight. Aim for a shallow squat at first, and gradually increase your depth as you become more comfortable. If necessary, use a sturdy chair behind you for support.

2. Wall Push-Ups: This modified version of traditional push-ups is excellent for building upper body strength without putting too much strain on your joints. Stand a few feet away from a wall and place your hands on the wall at shoulder height. Lean in towards the wall, then push back to the starting position. Repeat for several repetitions, adjusting your distance from the wall as needed to make it easier or more challenging.

Using Light Weights or Resistance Bands

Incorporating light weights or resistance bands into your routine can further enhance your strength training efforts. These tools allow you to perform a variety of exercises while maintaining a low impact on your joints.

1. Bicep Curls with Light Weights: Sit or stand comfortably with a light weight in each hand. Keep your elbows close to your body and curl the weights up towards your shoulders. Lower them back down with control. This exercise strengthens your arms and promotes joint stability in the elbows.

2. Resistance Band Rows: Anchor a resistance band at a low point (such as under a chair leg). Hold the ends of the band and sit with a straight back. Pull the band towards you while keeping your elbows close to your body, then slowly return to the starting position. This exercise targets the muscles in your back and shoulders, helping improve posture and stability.

Targeting Problem Areas: Knees, Wrists, Hips, and Shoulders

When designing a strength training routine, it's essential to target the areas most affected by arthritis. Exercises should focus on strengthening the muscles around these key joints to provide better support and alleviate discomfort.

1. Knee Strengthening: Leg raises are a great way to build strength without putting undue pressure on the knees. Sit on the edge of a chair with your feet flat on the ground. Extend one leg straight out in front of you and hold for a few seconds before lowering it back down. Alternate legs for several repetitions.

2. Wrist Strengthening: Wrist curls can help improve wrist stability. Sit comfortably with your forearm resting on your thigh, holding a light weight in your hand, palm facing up. Curl the weight up towards your body, then lower it back down. This simple movement can enhance strength in your wrists, crucial for daily activities.

3. Hip Strengthening: Side leg raises help target the muscles around the hips. Stand beside a wall or chair for support and lift one leg out to the side, keeping your body straight. Lower it back down and repeat on the other side.

4. Shoulder Strengthening: Overhead presses with light weights can build shoulder strength. Stand or sit with a weight in each hand, raise them to shoulder height, and then press upwards while maintaining a straight back. Return to shoulder height and repeat.

Best Practices for Safe Strength Training

While strength training is beneficial, it's essential to approach it with caution to avoid injury. Here are some best practices to keep in mind:

1. Avoiding Heavy Weights: It's vital to steer clear of heavy weights when starting your strength training journey. Heavy weights can place excessive strain on your joints and lead to injury. Instead, focus on light weights that allow for controlled movements.

2. Repetition and Form: When it comes to strength training, quality is far more important than quantity. Aim for 10 to 15 repetitions of each exercise, paying close attention to your form. Proper alignment and controlled movements help prevent injury and ensure you're effectively targeting the right muscles. If you're unsure about your form, consider working with a physiotherapist or trainer experienced in adaptive exercises.

3. Listening to Your Body: Finally, always listen to your body. If you experience pain or discomfort during any exercise, stop immediately. It's normal to feel some muscle fatigue, but sharp pain is a signal that something isn't right. Modify exercises as needed or consult with a healthcare professional to find alternatives that suit your abilities.

Strength training is an invaluable tool for individuals living with arthritis, providing essential support for weak joints and promoting overall health. By incorporating bodyweight exercises, light weights, and resistance bands into your routine, you can strengthen key areas while reducing the risk of injury.

As you embark on this strength training journey, remember to prioritize safety and listen to your body. Each small step you take contributes to greater stability, improved balance, and a more active lifestyle. With time, patience, and consistency, you'll discover the empowering effects of strength training, enhancing not only your physical health but also your confidence and overall well-being.

CHAPTER 5

FLEXIBILITY AND BALANCE TRAINING

Flexibility and balance are often overlooked components of a well-rounded fitness routine, yet they are essential, especially for those living with arthritis. In this chapter, we will delve into the importance of flexibility in managing arthritis, explore how yoga and Tai Chi can enhance joint health, and discuss practical modifications to ensure these practices remain accessible and beneficial.

Importance of Flexibility for Arthritis

Flexibility plays a crucial role in maintaining joint health and improving overall mobility. For individuals with arthritis, a greater range of motion can directly alleviate joint pain and stiffness, allowing for smoother movement throughout the day. Think of your joints as hinges on a door; if they don't have enough lubrication and flexibility, they'll creak and resist movement.

Take the case of Robert, a 72-year-old man diagnosed with rheumatoid arthritis. Robert struggled with daily tasks such as reaching for items on high shelves or bending down to tie his shoes. After starting a regular flexibility routine, he noticed significant improvements in his range of motion. Simple stretches allowed him to move with more ease, reducing the discomfort that had previously made his life challenging.

Maintaining flexibility over time is equally important. As we age, our bodies naturally lose some elasticity in muscles and tendons. Regular flexibility training helps counteract this decline, promoting joint health and enabling individuals with arthritis to stay active. By incorporating stretches into your daily routine, you can keep your joints supple and reduce the likelihood of stiffness, which often exacerbates pain.

Incorporating Yoga and Tai Chi

Two powerful practices that enhance flexibility and balance are yoga and Tai Chi. Both forms of exercise emphasize slow, controlled movements, making them particularly well-suited for individuals with arthritis.

Gentle Yoga Poses for Arthritis

Yoga offers a variety of poses that can be adapted for those with arthritis. Here are a few gentle poses to consider:

1. Child's Pose: This restorative pose stretches the back, hips, and thighs, providing gentle relief. Start on your hands and knees, then sit back on your heels and stretch your arms forward, resting your forehead on the ground. Breathe deeply and hold the pose for several breaths, allowing your body to relax.

2. Cat-Cow Stretch: This movement helps improve flexibility in the spine and releases tension in the back. Begin on all fours, with your wrists under your shoulders and your knees under your hips. Inhale as you arch your back, dropping your belly and lifting your head (the Cow Pose), and exhale as you round your back, tucking your chin to your chest (the Cat Pose). Repeat this cycle several times to increase mobility.

3. Seated Forward Bend: While sitting on the floor with your legs extended, slowly reach for your toes, allowing your back to round gently. If you can't reach your toes, that's okay! Simply rest your hands on your shins or thighs. This pose helps stretch the hamstrings and lower back, promoting flexibility in the hips and spine.

Benefits of Tai Chi

Tai Chi, often described as "meditation in motion," is another excellent practice for those with arthritis. It emphasizes slow, flowing movements, promoting balance, coordination, and relaxation. The gentle nature of Tai Chi makes it ideal for individuals with joint pain, as it minimizes impact while enhancing flexibility and strength.

Studies have shown that practicing Tai Chi can significantly improve balance and stability, which is crucial for reducing the risk of falls. For example, Janet, a 68-year-old woman with osteoarthritis in her knees, began attending a local Tai Chi class. Over time, she noticed not only improved balance but also a reduction in knee pain during her daily activities. The rhythmic movements of Tai Chi helped her feel more grounded and connected to her body.

Modifications for Arthritis-Friendly Poses and Movements

While yoga and Tai Chi are incredibly beneficial, it's essential to modify poses and movements to accommodate individual needs. Here are some helpful tips for making these practices more accessible:

1. Use Props: Yoga blocks, straps, and bolsters can provide extra support and help you maintain proper alignment. For instance, when performing a forward bend, a yoga block can be placed under your hands for added height and stability.

2. Listen to Your Body: Always pay attention to your body's signals. If a specific pose or movement causes pain, adjust your position or skip it altogether. Remember, there's no one-size-fits-all approach; find what feels best for you.

3. Start Slow: If you're new to yoga or Tai Chi, begin with shorter sessions and gradually increase the duration as you become more comfortable. Consistency is more important than intensity; aim for a few minutes each day to reap the benefits.

4. Consult a Teacher: If possible, seek out a qualified instructor experienced in working with individuals who have arthritis. They can offer valuable guidance on modifications and ensure you're practicing safely.

Incorporating flexibility and balance training into your fitness routine can significantly improve your quality of life if you have arthritis. Gentle yoga poses and the flowing movements of Tai Chi promote joint health, enhance mobility, and help reduce pain.

By embracing these practices, you can foster greater flexibility, stability, and a sense of well-being. As you continue your journey toward better health, remember that each gentle stretch and mindful movement contributes to a more active and fulfilling life. With patience and dedication, you'll discover the transformative effects of flexibility and balance training, enabling you to navigate the world with confidence and ease.

CHAPTER 6

CORE STRENGTH AND POSTURE IMPROVEMENT

Strengthening your core is about more than just building abdominal muscles; it's about enhancing the entire body's ability to support itself. For individuals with arthritis, a strong core can make a world of difference in how your body handles joint strain, especially in critical areas like the lower back and hips. In this chapter, we'll explore the importance of core strength for joint health and posture, as well as how to safely engage in core exercises that benefit people living with arthritis.

Why Core Strength is Important for Joint Health

Your core muscles include not just your abs but also the muscles in your lower back, hips, and pelvis. These muscles form the foundation of your body's stability, helping to distribute weight and reduce stress on your joints. Without a strong core, other parts of your body—like your knees, hips, or back—end up overcompensating, which can exacerbate arthritis symptoms.

A great example is Carol, a 55-year-old woman who suffered from osteoarthritis in her hips and lower back. Before focusing on her core, she often experienced pain and fatigue after standing for long periods. She noticed that her posture would slump, causing additional strain on her already sensitive joints. After beginning a gentle core strengthening routine, Carol found that her posture improved, and she experienced less discomfort in her hips and back. By strengthening her core, she distributed the load more evenly, helping her joints handle daily activities with less stress.

Reducing Joint Strain

When your core is strong, it acts like a stabilizer for your entire body. A well-supported core reduces unnecessary pressure on your joints by keeping your spine in alignment and your body balanced. For individuals with arthritis, this is especially important in areas like the lower back and hips, where poor posture or weak muscles can lead to further strain.

Think of your core as the anchor that holds everything together. Without this strong foundation, your joints can become overworked, leading to flare-ups or increased pain. Strengthening your core ensures that your body has the support it needs to handle movement, whether it's walking, lifting, or simply getting out of bed.

Improving Posture and Preventing Falls

Good posture is one of the key benefits of core strength. When your core is engaged, your body naturally aligns itself into a more stable position, reducing the chance of slumping or leaning into positions that might aggravate arthritis. Poor posture often leads to joint misalignment, which can exacerbate pain, especially in the spine, hips, and knees.

Strengthening your core also plays a significant role in preventing falls. Many people with arthritis experience a loss of balance due to joint stiffness or pain, which can increase the risk of falling. However, a strong core improves stability and coordination, making it easier to maintain balance during everyday activities. By building core strength, you're giving your body the tools it needs to move with more confidence and less risk of injury.

Core Exercises for Arthritis

Core exercises don't need to be strenuous to be effective. In fact, many low-impact core exercises can be performed seated or standing, reducing the strain on your joints while still engaging your muscles. The key is to focus on slow, controlled movements that activate your core without putting additional stress on your back or joints.

Here are some arthritis-friendly core exercises to consider:

Seated and Standing Core Exercises

1. Seated Torso Twist: Sit in a sturdy chair with your feet flat on the floor and your back straight. Slowly twist your torso to the right, keeping your hips square and facing forward. Hold for a few seconds, then return to the center. Repeat on the left side. This exercise strengthens your obliques while keeping pressure off your lower back and knees.

2. Standing Side Bends: Stand with your feet shoulder-width apart and your hands on your hips. Slowly bend to the right, sliding your right hand down the side of your thigh. Engage your core as you return to a standing position. Repeat on the left side. Side bends improve flexibility and strengthen the muscles along your sides, promoting better posture and reducing strain on your lower back.

Low-Impact Movements

1. Leg Lifts: Lie on your back with your knees bent and feet flat on the floor. Slowly lift one leg, keeping it bent at the knee, until your thigh is perpendicular to the floor. Lower it back down and repeat with the other leg. This exercise strengthens the lower abdominals without stressing the joints, making it ideal for those with arthritis in the hips or knees.

2. Modified Planks: Planks are excellent for core stability, but they can be hard on the wrists and shoulders for some people with arthritis. To modify, you can perform a plank on your knees instead of your toes, or even try a standing plank by leaning against a wall. Focus on keeping your core tight and your back straight while holding the position for 10-20 seconds, gradually increasing the duration as you get stronger.

3. Pelvic Tilts: Lie on your back with your knees bent and feet flat on the floor. Slowly tilt your pelvis upward, pressing your lower back into the floor as you engage your abdominal muscles. Hold for a few seconds, then release. This exercise helps strengthen the muscles in the lower abdomen and lower back, relieving pressure on the hips and promoting better posture.

Best Practices for Core Strengthening

While core strengthening exercises are beneficial, it's essential to approach them with care, especially if you're dealing with arthritis. Here are some tips to ensure you're practicing safely:

1. Start Slowly: If you're new to core exercises or haven't exercised in a while, start with a few repetitions and gradually increase as your strength improves. The goal is to challenge your muscles without causing discomfort.

2. Focus on Form: Maintaining proper form is more important than how many repetitions you can do. Poor form can strain your joints and exacerbate arthritis symptoms. Take your time with each movement, ensuring you're engaging your core without compromising other areas of your body.

3. Avoid Overexertion: Be mindful of how your body feels during and after exercise. It's normal to feel your muscles working, but you should never feel sharp or shooting pain. If you do, stop and reassess your form or consider modifying the exercise.

4. Stay Consistent: Consistency is key to building core strength. Aim to incorporate core exercises into your routine several times a week to see lasting improvements in your posture, balance, and joint health.

Strengthening your core is one of the most effective ways to support your joints and improve posture, especially if you're living with arthritis. By incorporating low-impact, arthritis-friendly core exercises into your routine, you can reduce strain on your joints, improve your balance, and stand tall with confidence. With time and dedication, you'll notice the benefits of a stronger core in your everyday life, allowing you to move more freely and comfortably.

CHAPTER 7

THE ROLE OF REST AND RECOVERY

In the journey of managing arthritis through exercise, rest and recovery often take a backseat to the more energetic aspects of a workout routine. However, understanding how to effectively integrate rest into your fitness regimen is crucial for long-term joint health and overall well-being. This chapter explores the importance of listening to your body, knowing when to rest, and implementing effective recovery strategies to help you feel your best after a workout.

Knowing When to Rest: Listening to Your Body

One of the most valuable skills you can develop as you engage in arthritis-friendly workouts is the ability to listen to your body. Pain is a natural signal that something may be wrong, but it's important to distinguish between pain that warrants immediate attention and discomfort that is part of the strengthening process.

Understanding Pain Versus Discomfort

For many individuals living with arthritis, the line between pain and discomfort can be blurred. Pain is often sharp and can indicate injury or excessive strain on your joints, while discomfort may feel like a dull ache or muscle fatigue after exercise. Learning to identify these differences can help you make informed decisions about when to push through a workout and when to take a break.

For instance, Linda, a 62-year-old woman with rheumatoid arthritis, initially struggled to differentiate between these sensations. After experiencing increased pain in her knees during a workout, she learned the importance of pausing and assessing her body's signals. By keeping a journal to track her workouts and how she felt afterward, Linda discovered that discomfort was manageable and temporary, while pain was a sign she needed to adjust her routine. This newfound awareness empowered her to make better choices about her exercise program.

Importance of Allowing Joints to Recover

Rest is just as critical as exercise in your fitness journey, especially for those with arthritis. Allowing your joints time to recover between workout sessions can help reduce inflammation and prevent flare-ups. This doesn't mean you need to stop moving altogether; rather, it's about giving specific muscles and joints the time they need to heal while still engaging in gentle activities that promote circulation and flexibility.

Incorporating rest days into your routine is essential. Depending on the intensity of your workouts, aim for at least one or two rest days each week. This time can be used for light activities, such as leisurely walks or gentle stretching, which keep your body engaged without overexerting your joints.

Post-Workout Recovery Tips

After completing your arthritis-friendly workouts, implementing effective recovery strategies can enhance your overall experience and ensure that you're ready for your next session. Here are some practical tips to help your joints recover:

Using Heat and Cold Therapy for Joint Pain Relief

Both heat and cold therapy can be invaluable tools in managing post-workout discomfort. Applying heat to sore muscles or stiff joints can help increase blood flow and relax tension. A warm bath, heating pad, or hot towel can provide soothing relief after a workout.

Conversely, cold therapy is beneficial for reducing inflammation and numbing sharp pain. Ice packs or cold compresses applied to affected joints can help minimize swelling and discomfort. Many individuals with arthritis find it helpful to alternate between heat and cold, depending on their specific symptoms.

For example, Mike, a 57-year-old man with osteoarthritis, discovered that using heat before his workouts helped warm up his stiff joints, making movement easier. After exercising, he would switch to cold therapy to soothe any inflammation, allowing him to feel more comfortable as he went about his day.

Incorporating Massage or Gentle Stretching to Reduce Stiffness

Massage can be a therapeutic way to promote recovery after your workouts. A professional massage therapist trained in working with arthritis patients can provide relief by targeting areas of tension and improving circulation. However, gentle self-massage techniques, such as using a foam roller or a massage ball, can also be effective in reducing stiffness and enhancing mobility.

In addition to massage, incorporating gentle stretching post-workout can help maintain flexibility and reduce muscle tension. Focus on stretches that target the major joints you've worked, holding each position for 15-30 seconds to encourage relaxation and ease stiffness.

Importance of Staying Hydrated and Maintaining Good Nutrition

Hydration and nutrition play critical roles in your recovery process. Dehydration can lead to increased joint pain and fatigue, so it's essential to drink plenty of water before, during, and after your workouts. Consider keeping a water bottle with you at all times to remind yourself to stay hydrated.

Equally important is the food you eat. A balanced diet rich in anti-inflammatory foods can support joint health and promote recovery. Incorporate plenty of fruits, vegetables, whole grains, lean proteins, and healthy fats into your meals. Foods rich in omega-3 fatty acids, such as salmon and walnuts, can help reduce inflammation, while antioxidants from colorful fruits and vegetables can combat oxidative stress.

For instance, Karen, a 65-year-old arthritis patient, noticed that after she adjusted her diet to include more anti-inflammatory foods, her overall joint pain diminished. By focusing on hydration and nutrition, she felt more energized and capable of completing her workouts without as much discomfort.

Rest and recovery are vital components of any successful arthritis-friendly workout routine. By learning to listen to your body, understanding the signals it sends, and incorporating effective recovery strategies, you can enhance your overall experience and maintain your joint health. Whether it's through heat and cold therapy, gentle stretching, or nourishing your body with the right foods, prioritizing recovery will enable you to continue engaging in physical activity with greater ease and comfort. Remember, a well-rested body is one that is ready to take on the next challenge, empowering you to live a healthier and more active life despite arthritis.

CHAPTER 8

MODIFYING EXERCISES BASED ON ARTHRITIS TYPE

Arthritis is not a one-size-fits-all condition. With various types affecting millions, customizing your exercise regimen to address specific needs is crucial for maintaining mobility and enhancing quality of life. In this chapter, we will explore how to tailor workouts based on whether you are dealing with osteoarthritis or rheumatoid arthritis. By understanding your unique condition, you can create an exercise routine that is both effective and safe, allowing you to stay active while protecting your joints.

Customizing Workouts for Osteoarthritis

Osteoarthritis (OA) is the most common form of arthritis, characterized by the degeneration of cartilage in the joints. As the protective cushion between bones wears down, it can lead to pain, stiffness, and reduced mobility. However, with the right approach, you can manage these symptoms while remaining active.

Joint-Specific Exercises for Knee, Hip, and Hand Osteoarthritis

When creating a workout plan for osteoarthritis, focusing on joint-specific exercises is essential. For those with knee OA, low-impact activities such as swimming or cycling can help strengthen the muscles around the knee without placing excessive strain on the joint. Additionally, exercises like leg lifts and seated marches can enhance quadriceps strength, providing better support for the knee.

For hip osteoarthritis, strength training is crucial. Targeted exercises like side leg lifts and clamshells can help stabilize the hip joint while maintaining flexibility. For those experiencing hand osteoarthritis, simple hand exercises—such as squeezing a stress ball or spreading fingers against resistance—can improve grip strength and overall dexterity.

While incorporating these exercises, it's important to be mindful of cartilage protection. Incorporating range-of-motion exercises, such as gentle stretching and yoga poses, can help maintain flexibility without causing undue stress. Always remember to warm up adequately before engaging in any activity to prepare your joints and muscles for movement.

Protecting Cartilage While Staying Active

Protecting cartilage is a priority when exercising with osteoarthritis. This means avoiding high-impact activities like running or jumping, which can exacerbate joint pain. Instead, choose exercises that promote low-impact movement and allow for gradual progression. Pay attention to your body's feedback—if an activity causes sharp pain or discomfort, modify or replace it with a gentler alternative.

Take, for example, Robert, a 58-year-old man with knee osteoarthritis. Initially, he was hesitant to engage in any physical activity, fearing it would worsen his condition. However, after consulting with a physiotherapist, he discovered a range of safe exercises tailored to his needs. By focusing on strengthening the muscles surrounding his knee through low-impact activities, Robert felt more confident and noticed a significant reduction in pain over time.

Customizing Workouts for Rheumatoid Arthritis

Rheumatoid arthritis (RA) presents a different set of challenges, as it is an autoimmune condition that can cause systemic inflammation and joint swelling. As such, managing inflammation while remaining active is key to maintaining joint function and overall health.

Managing Inflammation Through Low-Impact Movement

For individuals with RA, low-impact aerobic exercises—such as walking, cycling, or using an elliptical machine—can be beneficial. These activities help maintain cardiovascular health while minimizing strain on the joints. It's important to start slowly, gradually increasing duration and intensity based on how your body responds.

Additionally, incorporating flexibility and range-of-motion exercises can be highly advantageous. Gentle stretching and activities like yoga can improve joint mobility, enhance blood flow, and reduce stiffness. Poses such as Child's Pose or Cat-Cow can be particularly helpful, allowing for gentle movement that encourages relaxation and release of tension.

Adjusting Routines During Arthritis Flare-Ups

Flare-ups can occur unpredictably in rheumatoid arthritis, and it's essential to adapt your exercise routine accordingly. During periods of heightened inflammation, consider reducing the intensity of your workouts or opting for gentler activities. Swimming, for example, can be an excellent choice during a flare-up, as the buoyancy of the water alleviates pressure on the joints while providing a full-body workout.

In times of increased discomfort, active recovery techniques can also aid in managing symptoms. Gentle movements, such as stretching and slow walking, can maintain circulation without overexerting your joints. Take note of the importance of rest during flare-ups—allowing your body the time it needs to recover will ultimately support your long-term fitness goals.

One inspiring story comes from Jessica, a 44-year-old woman living with RA. During particularly challenging flare-ups, she learned to embrace restorative yoga as a way to maintain her practice. The gentle movements and deep breathing not only soothed her joints but also helped manage her stress levels. Jessica's journey illustrates the importance of adaptability in your fitness routine, empowering her to continue engaging in physical activity even when faced with challenges.

Understanding the differences between osteoarthritis and rheumatoid arthritis is essential for creating an effective exercise plan that addresses your specific needs. By customizing workouts to accommodate joint health, you can enhance your fitness journey while minimizing discomfort. Remember, whether you're focusing on joint-specific exercises for osteoarthritis or low-impact movement for rheumatoid arthritis, the key is to listen to your body and adjust your routine as needed. Your journey toward improved mobility and strength is uniquely yours, and with the right modifications, you can achieve your fitness goals while protecting your joints.

CHAPTER 9

STAYING MOTIVATED AND BUILDING A ROUTINE

Staying motivated to maintain a fitness routine can be challenging, especially for those dealing with the unpredictable nature of arthritis. However, with the right strategies and mindset, it's possible to build consistency and enjoy the journey toward better health. This chapter focuses on practical steps for establishing a routine, tracking progress, and connecting with supportive communities that can help you stay engaged in your fitness journey.

Building Consistency Without Overexertion

One of the fundamental aspects of a successful fitness routine is setting realistic goals. For individuals with arthritis, understanding your limitations and capabilities is essential to crafting a sustainable approach to exercise. Start by defining what you want to achieve—whether it's improving flexibility, increasing strength, or simply being more active. Setting specific, measurable, achievable, relevant, and time-bound (SMART) goals can help you focus on what's important without becoming overwhelmed.

For example, instead of aiming to run a marathon, consider setting a goal to walk for 15 minutes daily or complete two low-impact aerobics sessions each week. This approach allows you to build a consistent habit without the pressure of unrealistic expectations. As you accomplish these smaller goals, you'll find that your confidence grows, encouraging you to take on new challenges.

Overcoming mental blocks is also a crucial component of staying motivated. Fear of joint pain during exercise can create significant barriers to physical activity. To manage these fears, it's helpful to educate yourself about your condition and understand the benefits of exercise. Many people with arthritis find that engaging in physical activity can lead to reduced pain and increased mobility over time. Keeping this perspective in mind can help shift your focus from fear to empowerment.

Consider the journey of Karen, a 62-year-old woman who struggled with anxiety about exercising due to her knee osteoarthritis. Initially, she hesitated to start any routine, fearing that movement would exacerbate her pain. However, after gradually introducing low-impact activities, such as walking and stretching, she realized that not only could she move without discomfort, but she also felt a sense of accomplishment. By setting realistic goals and acknowledging her progress, Karen transformed her perspective on exercise from fear to excitement.

Tracking Progress and Celebrating Milestones

Monitoring your progress is vital for maintaining motivation. Keeping track of your activities can help you see how far you've come and identify areas for improvement. Fitness trackers, mobile apps, or even simple journals can provide a practical way to log your workouts and monitor your achievements. By documenting your routine, you can celebrate small victories, such as completing a certain number of workouts each week or achieving a specific stretch.

Celebrate every milestone, no matter how small. Did you manage to walk for 30 minutes instead of 20? Fantastic! Have you noticed that your flexibility has improved or your joint pain has decreased? Take a moment to recognize those achievements. Celebrating these wins reinforces your commitment to your fitness journey and encourages you to continue striving for improvement.

Maya, a 50-year-old woman with rheumatoid arthritis, embraced the power of tracking her progress through a fitness journal. Initially skeptical about her ability to maintain a routine, she started by recording her daily activities, including the time spent stretching and walking. As the weeks went by, she began to notice her gains in flexibility and energy levels. By acknowledging her progress in the journal, Maya built a positive feedback loop that kept her motivated to stay active.

Staying Connected with Supportive Communities

One of the most powerful motivators is connection with others. Joining arthritis-friendly fitness classes—whether in-person or online—can help you find a community of like-minded individuals who share similar challenges and goals. Participating in group classes not only provides structured workouts but also fosters a sense of camaraderie and support. You'll find encouragement from instructors and peers who understand your journey and can offer tips, share successes, and provide emotional support.

Additionally, connecting with support groups dedicated to arthritis can be incredibly beneficial. Many organizations offer resources and community forums where you can share experiences, seek advice, and celebrate achievements. Engaging with others who understand the complexities of living with arthritis can help you stay motivated and feel less isolated in your journey.

For example, David, a 47-year-old man with psoriatic arthritis, found his motivation to stay active through an online support group. By sharing his experiences with others, he discovered new exercise routines tailored for his needs and received encouragement from peers who were also navigating similar challenges. The sense of community not only kept him accountable but also inspired him to push through difficult days.

Staying motivated and building a consistent exercise routine is entirely achievable, even for those living with arthritis. By setting realistic goals, tracking your progress, and connecting with supportive communities, you can cultivate a fulfilling fitness journey. Remember that progress may not always be linear, but every small step you take toward your goals is significant. Embrace the process, celebrate your milestones, and lean on the support of others as you navigate the path to better health. Your commitment to staying active can lead to lasting improvements in your quality of life, paving the way for a more vibrant and fulfilling future.

CHAPTER 10

LIFESTYLE TIPS FOR LONG-TERM ARTHRITIS MANAGEMENT

Managing arthritis is not just about exercising; it involves a holistic approach that includes nutrition and daily habits. This chapter will explore how a mindful lifestyle, encompassing dietary choices and ergonomic adjustments, can significantly impact joint health and overall well-being.

The Role of Nutrition in Joint Health

The foods we consume play a pivotal role in managing arthritis symptoms. A diet rich in anti-inflammatory foods can help reduce pain and swelling, making it easier to stay active. Incorporating fruits, vegetables, whole grains, healthy fats, and lean proteins into your meals can support joint health. For example, berries, leafy greens, and fatty fish like salmon are packed with antioxidants and omega-3 fatty acids that combat inflammation.

Consider the story of Linda, a 55-year-old woman diagnosed with osteoarthritis. Initially skeptical about the impact of diet on her condition, she decided to consult a nutritionist. With guidance, Linda replaced processed foods with whole, nutrient-dense options. Her meals now include colorful salads, nuts, and seeds, which have not only enhanced her energy levels but also led to a noticeable decrease in her joint pain. After a few months of this dietary shift, she felt empowered to engage more actively in her workouts, illustrating how nutrition can be a game-changer for arthritis management.

Additionally, managing weight is crucial for individuals with arthritis, particularly for those with osteoarthritis. Excess weight adds pressure to weight-bearing joints, which can exacerbate pain and limit mobility. Establishing a balanced diet paired with regular physical activity can help maintain a healthy weight, alleviating strain on the joints. Small, manageable changes in daily eating habits—like swapping sugary snacks for healthier options—can lead to significant improvements over time.

Creating a Joint-Friendly Daily Routine

Integrating movement into your daily life doesn't have to be complicated. Simple adjustments can make a big difference in how you feel. For instance, standing up and stretching during long periods of sitting can help keep your joints flexible and reduce stiffness. Taking short walks during breaks or choosing to park further away from your destination are easy ways to incorporate more movement into your day.

Maya, a 62-year-old retiree, discovered that creating a joint-friendly daily routine was key to managing her arthritis. She began by setting reminders on her phone to stand up and stretch every hour while working at her desk. Additionally, she incorporated walking her dog into her daily schedule, turning it into a delightful bonding experience that also allowed her to get some fresh air and exercise. These small changes not only helped her maintain flexibility but also provided mental breaks that improved her overall well-being.

Ergonomic adjustments in your home and workspace can also enhance joint comfort and reduce strain. For example, using a chair with good lumbar support, positioning your computer screen at eye level, or using tools designed for ease of grip can make everyday tasks more manageable. If you spend a lot of time in the kitchen, consider investing in adaptive utensils that require less force to use, or place frequently used items within easy reach to minimize unnecessary bending or stretching.

John, a 58-year-old office worker, struggled with wrist pain due to prolonged typing. After consulting an ergonomic specialist, he made several changes to his workspace. He switched to a keyboard with a softer touch and raised his chair to ensure his wrists remained straight while typing. As a result, John experienced less discomfort and was able to focus better on his work, demonstrating how thoughtful adjustments can lead to significant improvements in daily life.

Incorporating nutrition and lifestyle modifications into your daily routine is vital for effective long-term arthritis management. By choosing anti-inflammatory foods and maintaining a healthy weight, you can alleviate some of the pressure on your joints. Additionally, integrating more movement into your day and making ergonomic adjustments can enhance your comfort and overall quality of life. Remember, managing arthritis is a journey that requires a multifaceted approach. By making these lifestyle changes, you can empower yourself to lead a more active and fulfilling life, proving that arthritis doesn't have to define your journey. Embrace these tips, and take charge of your health—one small step at a time.

CONCLUSION

Living with arthritis does not mean sacrificing an active lifestyle; rather, it provides an opportunity to redefine what fitness means to you. Embracing a positive mindset towards exercise can transform your journey from one of limitations to one filled with potential. Instead of focusing on what you can't do, it's crucial to recognize and celebrate what you can achieve. Each small step taken toward fitness is a testament to your strength and resilience.

Consider the stories shared throughout this book—individuals who have navigated the challenges of arthritis by adapting their workouts and embracing their bodies' capabilities. Their journeys remind us that staying active is not about perfection; it's about progress. Whether it's a gentle walk in the park, a refreshing swim, or a short session of stretching, every effort counts. Staying committed to arthritis-friendly workouts can lead to long-term rewards, including improved joint health, enhanced mood, and a greater sense of independence.

The journey toward managing arthritis is uniquely personal, and it is filled with ups and downs. Yet, maintaining a commitment to an active lifestyle can have profound benefits, not only for physical health but also for emotional well-being. As you continue to explore and implement the strategies discussed in this book, remember that every movement matters. You have the power to create a life filled with activity and joy, regardless of your arthritis.

Appendices

Arthritis-Friendly Workout Plan for Beginners

To help you get started, here is a sample weekly schedule for low-impact exercises that you can adapt based on your preferences and abilities:

Weekly Schedule:

Day	Activity	Duration
Monday	Gentle Walking	20-30 min
Tuesday	Water Aerobics	30 min
Wednesday	Rest Day or Light Stretching	10-15 min
Thursday	Chair-Based Aerobics	20-30 min
Friday	Cycling (Stationary or Outdoor)	30 min
Saturday	Yoga or Tai Chi (Gentle Flow)	30 min
Sunday	Rest Day or Leisurely Walk	20-30 min

Feel free to modify this schedule to fit your lifestyle. The key is to incorporate variety and listen to your body, ensuring that you remain comfortable while challenging yourself.

Resources and Further Reading

To support your journey, here are some valuable resources for arthritis-friendly fitness tips and information:

Websites:

- Arthritis Foundation: [www.arthritis.org] (http://www.arthritis.org)

- Mayo Clinic: [www.mayoclinic.org] (http://www.mayoclinic.org)

- American College of Rheumatology: [www.rheumatology.org] (http://www.rheumatology.org)

Books:

- "The Arthritis Foundation's Guide to Good Living with Arthritis" by the Arthritis Foundation

- "Eat to Beat Arthritis: The 5-Step Program for Pain-Free Living" by Dr. David S. Felten

Organizations:

- Arthritis Foundation: Provides resources, support, and community events.

- Local gyms or community centers: Many offer specialized arthritis-friendly fitness classes.

As you continue to explore the world of fitness and arthritis, remember that you are not alone. There is a community of support available, and together, we can thrive while managing arthritis. Embrace your journey with an open heart, and know that a vibrant, active life awaits you!